Mona BOUDABBOUS
Marwa BOUJELBENE

ANEMIA AND CHRONIC INFLAMMATORY BOWEL DISEASE

Mona BOUDABBOUS
Marwa BOUJELBENE

ANEMIA AND CHRONIC INFLAMMATORY BOWEL DISEASE

What to do in practice?

ScienciaScripts

Imprint
Any brand names and product names mentioned in this book are subject to trademark, brand or patent protection and are trademarks or registered trademarks of their respective holders. The use of brand names, product names, common names, trade names, product descriptions etc. even without a particular marking in this work is in no way to be construed to mean that such names may be regarded as unrestricted in respect of trademark and brand protection legislation and could thus be used by anyone.

Cover image: www.ingimage.com

This book is a translation from the original published under ISBN 978-620-6-68976-8.

Publisher:
Sciencia Scripts
is a trademark of
Dodo Books Indian Ocean Ltd. and OmniScriptum S.R.L publishing group

120 High Road, East Finchley, London, N2 9ED, United Kingdom
Str. Armeneasca 28/1, office 1, Chisinau MD-2012, Republic of Moldova, Europe
Printed at: see last page
ISBN: 978-620-6-59925-8

INTRODUCTION

Inflammatory bowel disease (IBD), which mainly includes Crohn's disease (CD) and ulcerative colitis (UC), is a chronic condition characterised by chronic inflammation of the intestine, with flare-ups interspersed with periods of remission (1,(2). Their aetiopathogenesis is multifactorial, involving a genetic predisposition, an inappropriate immune response and environmental factors (3),(4),(5).

Clinically, intestinal manifestations are often in the foreground. However, a wide range of extra-intestinal symptoms can also occur during the course of the disease. Anemia is in fact the most common extra-intestinal manifestation of IBD (6). Its frequency varies between 6 and 74% depending on the series (7).

According to the European Crohn's and Colitis Organisation (ECCO) guidelines, anaemia in IBD patients can be classified as iron deficiency anaemia, inflammatory anaemia, mixed anaemia and anaemia associated with vitamin B12 or folic acid deficiency (3),(8,9). However, since IBD patients present with concomitant chronic intestinal bleeding, inflammation, reduced absorption, malnutrition, and possible toxic effects of drugs and surgery, the exact aetiology of the anaemia cannot be determined. Its pathogenesis is therefore generally multifactorial (9). Furthermore, anaemia in IBD significantly affects patients' quality of life and work, and increases the number of hospital admissions. It thus generates additional healthcare costs (2),(3).

Effective treatment of anaemia in IBD patients has been shown to significantly improve their quality of life.

of life (10). It is therefore necessary to understand the pathophysiological mechanisms of anaemia in these patients and to identify the main risk factors in order to ensure appropriate, targeted management.

In this context, the objectives of this book are :

- specify the characteristics of anaemia in patients with IBD;
- and to look for any factors associated with the onset and persistence of anaemia in IBD patients.

In a review of 22 articles, the mean prevalence of anaemia in IBD patients was 17% (95% CI: 16-18) (17). In a meta-analysis, the prevalence of anaemia in 2192 IBD patients was 24% (27% in CD patients and 21% in UC patients) (18). Although anaemia is the most frequent complication and extraintestinal manifestation of inflammatory bowel disease, its exact mechanism is often poorly understood in these patients due to its multifactorial nature. However, its impact on patients' quality of life is well established, with a reduction in both physical and intellectual performance (2) (10). What's more, anaemia can occasionally appear before the digestive signs of IBD, thus inaugurating the diagnosis (10),(19). For all these reasons, we carried out this study with the aim of defining the characteristics of anaemia in patients with inflammatory bowel disease and identifying possible risk factors for its occurrence and persistence, in order to target patients at risk and optimise their management and monitoring.

CHAPTER I. MAIN MECHANISMS OF ANEMIA IN MICI

As found in a study carried out in our centre (see last chapter), the types of anaemia most frequently encountered in IBD are primarily iron deficiency anaemia and inflammatory anaemia (20). Anemias due to vitamin B12 and folate deficiencies are not uncommon in IBD patients. There are also rare causes of anaemia such as drug-induced anaemia, haemolytic anaemia and anaemia associated with myelodysplasia.

Iron deficiency anaemia can be caused by intestinal haemorrhage, insufficient absorption (inflammatory areas of the duodenum and jejunum), chronic inflammation of the intestine (impact on absorption, transport and storage of iron) and reduction in the amount of iron in the diet (dietary restriction or habit) (21),(22). In the literature, the frequency of anaemia due to iron deficiency varies between 17.6% and 29.9% (6),(23). However, it is important to specify that the assessment of martial status in these studies was very heterogeneous in terms of methodology (Table XXVII). In our work, a deficiency origin was immediately assumed when ferritinemia was plummeted (< 30 pg/ml). In the other cases (normal or elevated ferritin), we took into account the serum C-reactive protein level to distinguish between pure inflammatory anaemia and mixed anaemia in accordance with ECCO recommendations (11). Our approach was justified by the fact that ferritin levels may be falsely normal or even increased in the presence of an inflammatory syndrome.

In several studies, the soluble transferrin receptor (RsTf) has been identified as a highly specific diagnostic tool for martial deficiency. In the literature, several studies have investigated variations in RsTf levels as a function of martial status, as well as its contribution to the differential diagnosis between pure iron deficiency anaemia and anaemia of chronic inflammatory diseases(24-26). Unfortunately, our study did not investigate this marker, as its use in current practice is limited by its high cost. Inflammatory anaemia caused by chronic inflammation is mainly due to cytokines, which reduce plasma iron levels and subsequently its bioavailability for erythropoiesis. In addition, inflammatory cytokines have a direct inhibitory effect on erythropoiesis, which also contributes to the development of anaemia (27),(26). Iron-deficiency and inflammatory anaemia may be associated, resulting in mixed anaemia (6). The mechanism of anaemia due to vitamin B12 or folate deficiency is complex. It depends on the type of IBD. Crohn's disease (CD) is a chronic inflammatory disease that frequently involves the terminal ileum, which is the site of vitamin B12 absorption. Long-term inflammation of this mucosa can lead to impaired absorption, fibrosis and also strictures that require surgical resection of segments of the intestine including the ileum. Subsequently, CD patients are particularly at risk of vitamin B12 deficiency. In contrast, although UC is also an inflammatory bowel disease, it is limited to the colon, without ileal involvement, and therefore the prevalence of B12 deficiency in UC patients is similar to the general prevalence [28]. However, in our study, 4 of 28 patients (14.3%) were vitamin B12 deficient. This frequency was higher than in two studies in the literature where vitamin B12 deficiency was 1.5% and 5% during IBD (10,23). In addition, only 1 of our 4 patients had Crhon's disease. This discrepancy with the data in the literature is probably due to the relatively small size of our sample and the high frequency of UC in our series (Table XXVII).

Table I: Frequency of each type of anaemia in IBD according to studies

<table>
<tr><th rowspan="2">Authors</th><th rowspan="2">Definition used</th><th rowspan="2">N</th><th colspan="5">Frequency of anaemia (%)</th></tr>
<tr><th colspan="2">Total</th><th colspan="2">IDA</th><th>ACD</th></tr>
<tr><td>Bengi G et al (6)</td><td>IDA: ferritin < 30pg/l and transferrin <20%.
CDA: ferritin > 100pg/l and transferrin <20%.</td><td>465</td><td colspan="2">51.6</td><td colspan="2">29.9</td><td>8</td></tr>
<tr><td rowspan="2">Akhuemonkhan et al(8)</td><td rowspan="2">IDA: (ferritin<30pg/l) or (ferritin<100 and high CRP)</td><td rowspan="2">669</td><td>CD</td><td>RCH</td><td>CD</td><td>RCH</td><td rowspan="2"></td></tr>
<tr><td>32,4</td><td>27,6</td><td>9,2</td><td>85,1</td></tr>
<tr><td>Goodhand et al(29)</td><td>IDA: (ferritin<30pg/l) or [ferritin<100 and (CRP >10) or (transferrin<16%)].
CDA: ferritin > 100pg/l and transferrin <16%.</td><td>124</td><td colspan="2">40</td><td colspan="2">55</td><td>27</td></tr>
<tr><td>Özlen et al (30)</td><td>IDA: ferritin < 30pg/l and transferrin <20%.
CDA: ferritin > 100pg/l and transferrin <20%.</td><td>201</td><td colspan="2">58.2</td><td colspan="2">59.7</td><td>4.9</td></tr>
</table>

IDA: iron deficiency anaemia; ACD: inflammatory anaemia; CD: Crohn's disease; N: total number of patients in the study

CHAPTER II. MARTIAL DEFICIENCY IN NON-ANAEMICS

Martial deficiency is the most common nutritional deficiency in the world, particularly in IBD patients (31),(32),(33). It is a major precipitating factor in anaemia. In fact, the high concentrations of inflammatory cytokines found in patients with chronic inflammatory diseases increase hepcidin concentrations, leading to iron sequestration in the cells of the reticuloendothelial system (functional iron deficiency). Generally, assays to assess iron stores are only requested in the context of anaemia, however martial deficiency, even without anaemia, is present in approximately half of patients with chronic inflammatory diseases (32).

Ferritin is a sensitive indicator for detecting martial deficiency (34),(35). In current practice, martial deficiency is defined as a ferritin level of less than 30 pg/L. Since ferritin is an indicator of inflammation, which increases during chronic inflammatory states, the ferritin threshold values for defining martial deficiency are increased to 100 pg/L in states of chronic inflammation (31). This definition has been adopted by the ECCO (32). Unfortunately, there is no consensual practical guide in the literature that defines martial deficiency independently of anaemia due to martial deficiency, particularly in IBD.

Soluble transferrin receptor (RsTf) is also useful for diagnosing martial deficiency. It is mainly used when ferritinaemia is between 100 pg/l and 300 pg/l (in chronic inflammatory states), as it does not increase in chronic inflammatory states, unlike ferritinaemia (31). As mentioned above, this marker was not used in our study due to its high cost. Serum iron measurement is not recommended for the diagnosis of martial deficiency as its levels fluctuate throughout the day (31,36).

On reviewing the literature, we found that the frequency of martial deficiency varied considerably between studies, with extremes ranging from 13% to 90% (32),(37),(38). The great variability in this frequency can be explained, at least in part, by the heterogeneity of the populations studied. On the other hand, the difference between the definitions adopted for martial deficiency may also explain the wide range of frequencies of martial deficiency reported in the literature. Steint et al estimate that one third of patients with martial deficiency without anaemia will subsequently develop anaemia (38). According to Benjamin et al, approximately 14% of non-anaemic IBD patients were martially deficient, with no significant difference between Crohn's disease and UC patients. However, in this study, martial deficiency was defined as a ferritin level below 20 pg/l or a transferrin level above 28 mg/l (39).

CHAPTER III. RISK FACTORS FOR ANEMIA IN MICI

3.1. Risk factors common to the different types of anaemia

3.1.1. Localisation of IBD

In our study (see last chapter), UC patients with pan-colonic disease had a higher risk of developing anaemia than those with less extensive UC. This result is consistent with the literature, where the frequency of anaemia increases with the extent of the disease (30),(9),(40).

For Crohn's disease, the data in the literature are discordant. In fact, as in our study, Antunes CV et al found that the different locations of Crohn's disease had no influence on the risk of anaemia (10). On the other hand, in the study by Foteinogiannopoulou K et al, ileal location was a risk factor for developing anaemia and ileocolic location appeared to be less frequent in patients who had never developed anaemia. While Wozniak et al showed that anaemia was frequent in patients with ileocolic Crohn's disease (70.96% vs. 56.52%, with ; p = 0.03) (40).

3.1.2. Rate of hospitalisation

In our study, the rate of hospitalisations was higher in the anaemic group, with a significant difference (p<0.0001) for both UC and Crohn's disease patients. This result is consistent with data from two series published in 2009 and 2021 (31,33). It is to be expected, given that anaemia is one of the criteria for the severity of IBD attacks, requiring patients to be hospitalised. Moreover, in our study, 45.6% of anaemic UC patients had a severe inaugural flare versus no non-anaemic patients, while 70% of non-anaemic patients had a minimal inaugural flare versus 38.5% (p<0.0001). This result is also explained by the fact that in the majority of our patients, anaemia was discovered during the inaugural attack. Such an association has not been specifically investigated in the literature.

3.1.3. Abdominal pain

Abdominal pain was more frequent in anaemic patients in our study ($p=0.025$). This association has not been specifically investigated in the literature. However, several studies in the literature have established a relationship between this symptom and inflammation or disease activity (41),(42),(43). Moreover, abdominal pain is one of the indices used to assess disease activity, such as the Lichtiger score and the CDAI score (13) (Appendix 7).

3.1.4. Body mass index

In our study, overweight was more common among non-anaemic patients (50%) than anaemic patients (22.5%), with a significant difference ($p=0.011$). This result is consistent with the fact that both BMI and haemoglobin levels are parameters for assessing the nutritional status of patients in general, including patients with IBD. This result is found in the literature. In the study by Foteinogiannopoulouet K et al, the mean BMI of patients who had never developed anaemia was higher than that of patients who developed anaemia during the course of their IBD ($p=0.0001$). In another study, the authors concluded that patients with active IBD had a lower BMI than control patients with inactive IBD. Furthermore, in the same study, mean haemoglobin and ferritin levels in these patients were lower than in control patients (44).

3.1.5. WHO score

A WHO score greater than 0 was more frequent in anaemic patients, with a significant difference (p=0.001) attesting to a more frequently altered general condition in these patients. This association has not been specifically investigated in the literature, but this result seems logical since anaemia can alter general condition through the asthenia it generates.

3.1.6. Hypoalbuminemia

In our study, 60% of our anaemic patients had hypoalbuminemia compared with 25% of non-anaemic patients, with a statistically significant difference (p=0.002). This result is consistent with the literature. In the study by wozinak et al, a positive correlation was found between serum albumin and haemoglobin levels in both types of IBD, with $p<0.05$ (40). Furthermore, in another more recent study, a serum albumin level of less than 33g/l was predictive of moderate or severe anaemia in patients with Crohn's disease (45). Serum albumin decreases in inflammatory states as a result of increased vascular permeability, increased renal clearance and altered hepatic synthesis (46).

Hypoalbuminemia is generally attributed to malnutrition, but malnutrition does not result in significant and profound hypoalbuminemia in the absence of inflammation (46). In IBD, the cause of low serum albumin may also be multifactorial, resulting from systemic inflammation, malnutrition or both (9),(47).

3.1.7. Serum CRP level

A serum CRP level > 6 mg/l was a risk factor associated with the development of anaemia in our patients. In fact, CRP is an objective marker of acute inflammation that is strongly associated with anaemia. This finding confirms the importance of inflammation in the pathophysiology of anaemia in

IBD (48). Its elevation in the context of uncomplicated IBD is often associated with a relapse of the disease.

This result was found in a study in which serum CRP levels were higher in anaemic patients than in non-anaemic patients during the course of 2 types of IBD ($p<0.001$ for patients with Crohn's disease and $p=0.009$ for patients with UC). In this series, the risk of anaemia increased by 90% for each 1 mg/l rise in CRP in the univariate analysis (10). In another series, mean serum CRP level was negatively correlated with haemoglobin level with a significant difference for Crohn's disease only ($p=0.002$ for Crohn's disease patients, $p=0.07$ for UC patients) (40).

3.1.8. Systemic corticosteroid therapy

Our anaemic patients had more frequent recourse to systemic corticosteroids during one of the relapses occurring after the onset of anaemia ($p=0.025$). The same result was observed in the study by Göksel et al, where patients who received corticosteroid-based treatment developed more anaemia (6). Corticosteroids have been used to induce remission in UC and Crohn's disease since the 1950s (49). However, the data in the literature on their association with the presence of anaemia is sparse and inconsistent. In a Korean study, anaemia was associated with oral corticosteroid therapy in a male population with UC. However, in this study, there was no relationship between the use of intravenous corticosteroids and anaemia (50).

Treatment with immunosuppressants

In our population, 52.5% of anaemic patients were on immunosuppressants compared with 12.5% of non-anaemic patients ($p<0.0001$). Several studies have found the same result as our study (31,45,13,3). Immunosuppressants are generally used as a second-line treatment for moderate to severe forms of UC, resistant forms, corticosteroid-dependent forms and recurrent forms. They currently represent the validated first-line maintenance treatment for Crohn's disease (51). In addition, thiopurine may cause normocytic normochromic anaemia because it induces megaloblastic anaemia. In addition, the combination of microcytic anaemia due to iron deficiency and macrocytosis induced by azathioprine may lead to normocytic normochromic anaemia (50).

Among our anaemic patients, only one was put on methotrexate. This treatment was discontinued 2 months after the onset of his anaemia. Such an association has not been specifically investigated in the literature in IBD patients, but the haematological toxicity of methotrexate is well known (52). Indeed, patients treated with methotrexate may experience haematological adverse events, including myelosuppression, leukopenia, neutropenia and megaloblastic anaemia (52),(53). In our patient, the drug-induced origin of the anaemia is uncertain since the anaemia appeared 2 months before the metheroxate was taken. However, the anaemia disappeared one month after the start of this treatment.

3.1.9. Treatment with anti-TNF a

Anemia is associated with the use of anti-TNF **a** during IBD in series published in the literature (9),(50).

Anti-TNF **a** drugs are one of the treatments used in IBD to achieve remission and prevent relapses (54). In the literature, they are not incriminated in the onset of anaemia, but rather in the development of opportunistic infections and heart failure (55),(56).

Anti-TNF **a** drugs are mainly indicated in moderate to severe forms of IBD after other alternatives have failed (57),(58). These active forms are more frequently associated with anaemia (50),(9),(6).

In our sample, only one patient was treated with anti-TNF **a drugs**. He had anaemia.

3.1.10. Gender

In IBD, the percentage of anaemic women was higher than that of non-anaemic women (9),(6),(23),(40),(59). In the study by Koutroubakis IE, the prevalence of anaemia during IBD was higher in women, with a more remarkable difference in young women. Given the bleeding during menstruation and the higher frequency of IBD in young women, the increase in anaemia in these women is plausible (23).

3.1.11. Type of IBD

L ost series in the literature have shown that anaemia is more frequent in patients with Crohn's disease than in those with UC (2),(48),(9),(18),(19). This is probably related to extensive and/or stenosing bowel involvement in their Crohn's disease patients resulting in malabsorption with undernutrition probably associated with food intolerance and/or self-restriction.

3.1.12. Heart rate

Our study showed that anaemic patients had a higher mean heart rate than our non-anaemic patients, with a statically significant difference (p=0.013). This result is expected since anaemia increases heart rate (7). In addition, a heart rate greater than 90 beats/min is a sign of severity in advanced IBD and forms part of the Truelove score (60).

3.2. Risk factors for persistent and/or recurrent anaemia :

The evolution of the anaemia in our patients was marked by its disappearance in 45% of patients compared with its persistence and/or recurrence in the remainder (see last chapter). Our results are comparable with those of the study by Foteinogiannopoulou K et al. In this study, 29.6% of patients showed disappearance of anaemia with a study period estimated at 1 year (31). The search for risk factors for persistence and/or recurrence of anaemia is imperative, given that recurrent/persistent anaemia is strongly correlated with the most severe and disabling forms of IBD (61).

Comparing anaemic patients according to the evolution of their anaemia (disappearance versus persistence and/or recurrence), we found that the group with persistent and/or recurrent anaemia had a significantly lower initial haemoglobin level than the group with disappearance of the anaemia (p=0.016). In addition, the mean age was significantly lower in patients with persistent/recurrent anaemia (41.04±14.67 years versus 50.77±10.81 years). respectively, **p=0.025**). This result may be explained by more severe disease in younger patients. Finally, patients with persistent and/or recurrent anaemia had more glairosanguineous diarrhoea than patients with improved anaemia (86.4% versus 55.6%, **p=0.04**).

In the literature, these factors were not found. However, the factors predictive of persistent and/or recurrent anaemia in IBD patients varied from study to study. In the study by Foteinogiannopoulou K et al, persistent and/or recurrent anaemia was associated with Crohn's disease, a longer duration of the disease, surgery, a high number of hospital admissions, treatment with anti TNF **a drugs** and extra digestive manifestations (9). However, in another study, these factors were the number of hospitalisations, the number of gastrology consultations, history of surgery, high CRP levels and finally elevated blood sedimentation rate (61). On the other hand, in a study carried out on a paediatric population, the authors did not find any factors predictive of persistence and/or recurrence of anaemia (45).

CHAPTER IV. TREATMENT OF ANEMIA

Patients' quality of life improves with correction of anaemia, and this improvement is independent of disease activity (22). The European Consensus Conference recommends correcting anaemia in IBD when it is detected. However, the correction of martial deficiency without anaemia remains a subject of controversy, depending on patients' history, symptoms and preferences (20) (22). According to ECCO recommendations, the aim of treatment is to normalise haemoglobin levels and iron stores (22). The acceptable rate of correction of anaemia is either an increase in haemoglobin of at least 2 g/dl, or its normalisation within 4 weeks. This is the marker for therapeutic efficacy (22).

Haemoglobin levels in IBD patients must always be monitored, given the high incidence of anaemia and its major impact on patients' quality of life (22) .

Treatment of IBD is an important measure for correcting anaemia (62).

Management of anaemia in IBD involves several therapeutic approaches:

4.1. Oral martial therapy

The majority of our patients (96.4%) who received treatment for their anaemia received oral supplementation Oral iron is generally prescribed by physicians because of its lower cost, non-invasive route, ease of administration and established safety profile (7).Despite these advantages, its indications remain limited in IBD patients.

According to the ECCO, oral iron is indicated for patients with moderate anaemia, clinically inactive IBD and no intolerance to this treatment.

Orally administered iron is only partially absorbed and unabsorbed iron salts can be toxic to the intestinal mucosa.

High doses can also aggravate inflammation, as non-adsorbed salts appear to have a pro-inflammatory action (22).

The dose of elemental iron recommended by the ECCO should not exceed 100 mg/d for adults and 2-3mg/kg/d for children (7) .

4.2. Intravenous martial therapy :

In our series, of the anaemic patients who received treatment for their anaemia, 21.4% received intravenous martial therapy. The treatment received was based on ferric sucrose hydroxide (Veinofer®).

The usual treatment of iron deficiency anaemia with oral iron has its limitations in IBD patients. In fact, intravenous iron is a very good therapeutic alternative. It is more effective, faster and much better tolerated (22).

Three different generations of intravenous iron are available:

- The first generation is mainly iron dextran with a high molecular weight,
- The second generation, mainly iron gluconate and iron sucrose
- And finally the $3^{éme}$ generation represented by fermoxytol, iron carboxymaltose and iron isomaltoside (7).

The first generation of intravenous iron has been abandoned because of the high risk of developing anaphylactic shock.

According to the ECCO, intravenous iron is indicated in patients with clinically active IBD, ACTD of oral iron intolerance, haemoglobin levels below 10g/l and finally erythropoietin treatment (22).

4.3. Agents stimulating erythropoiesis

The use of erythropoietin (EPO) in the treatment of anaemia in IBD should be reserved for patients with severe, symptomatic anaemia refractory to IV iron supplementation, who would require blood transfusions and for whom aggressive disease-modifying therapy (immunosuppressants, anti-TNF, etc.) has failed to reduce mucosal inflammation (20).

In our study, no patient had received this treatment. This treatment is not in common practice given its high cost and potentially serious adverse effects (20).

The efficacy of erythropoiesis-stimulating agents is limited by concomitant functional iron deficiency. This is why they are used in combination with intravenous iron (20).

4.4. Blood transfusions

Transfusion in IBD patients should be limited and reserved for special situations (haemoglobin level below 7 g/l, severe acute anaemia, anaemia with haemodynamic instability and failure of other treatments) (22). According to ECCO recommendations, transfusion should be associated with martial supplementation (22).

In our study, five patients (17.9%) received a blood transfusion. All had haemoglobin levels below 8.5g/l.

4.5. Controlling inflammation

Of the anaemic patients, 12 had received neither martial therapy nor transfusion; 66.6% of these patients had improved anaemia.

The disappearance of anaemia in these patients is probably due to the control of systemic inflammation.

According to the ECCO, the main treatment for inflammatory anaemia is to achieve complete remission of IBD (22).

4.6. Dietary advice and adaptation

Increasing the amount of iron-rich foods can help maintain iron stores at an appropriate level (3).

CHAPTER V. RESULTS OF A SINGLE-CENTRE STUDY

Our study population consisted of 80 patients with IBD attending the gastroenterology outpatient clinic at the Hédi Chaker University Hospital, Sfax: 40 patients with anaemia versus 40 patients without anaemia. Among our patients, 57 had UC (71.3%) and 23 had Crohn's disease (28.7%).

5.1. Descriptive study

5.1.1. Socio-demographic characteristics of IBD patients

The average age of patients was 47.97 ±14.66 years, with extremes ranging from 18 to 80 years.

The mean age of anaemic patients was 45.43±3.81 years compared with 50.63±13.81 years, with a non-significant difference (p=0.122).

Of the IBD patients, 55% were women, with an M/F sex ratio of 0.82.

5.1.2. Personal history of proton pump inhibitor use

Of our 80 patients, 13 (16.3%) had a history of PPI use lasting more than 6 months.

5.1.3. Family history of IBD

Among our patients, 5 (6.3%) had a family history of IBD. These patients all had anaemia. The relationship was 1 degree in one patient, 2 degrees in 3 patients and 3 degrees in one patient.

None of the patients in our sample had a history of resection of the last ileal loop or extensive resection of the small bowel.

5.1.4. Lifestyle habits

Among our patients, 15 (18.8%) were smokers and 4 (5%) consumed alcohol.

5.1.5. Characteristics of the disease

In our sample, 57 patients had UC and 23 had Crohn's disease.

5.1.5.1. Crohn's disease (CD)

Of the 23 patients with Crohn's disease, 13 (52.17%) developed anaemia compared with 11 (47.83%) without anaemia.

The most common site of Crohn's disease was ileocolic (60.9%), followed by ileal (30.4%). Anoperineal lesions were found in 17.4% of cases. No patient had proximal gastrointestinal tract involvement. Crohn's disease was non-stenotic and non-fistulising in 17 patients (73.9%) (Table II).

Table II: Distribution of our population according to the phenotypic classification of Montreal Crohn's disease

		N total =23		*With anaemia (n=13)*		*No anaemia(n=10)*	
		Workforce	*%*	*Workforc*	*%*	*Workforce*	*%*
Crohn's A	Al	3	13	2	15,4	1	10
	A2	14	60,9	8	61,5	6	60
	A3	6	26,1	3	23,1	3	30
Crohn's L	L1 ileal	7	30,4	3	23,1	4	40
	L2 colonic	2	8,7	1	7,7	1	10
	L3 ileocolic	14	60,9	9	69,2	5	50
Crohn's B	B1 non-stenosing non-fistulising	17	73,9	9	69,2	8	80
	B2 stenosis	3	13	2	15,4	1	10
	B3 fistulising	3	13	2	15,4	1	10
	p (anoperineal lesions)	4	17,4	2	15,2	2	20

The inaugural attack of Crohn's disease was judged to be minimal according to the CDAI score in more than half the cases, and moderate in about a third (Table II).

None of the patients with Crohn's disease in our sample had had a severe inaugural attack.

Table III: Classification of patients with Crohn's disease according to the CDAI score at the time of the inaugural attack

	n=23	
	Workforce	*%*
Not active	3	13
Minimal activity	12	52,2
Moderate activity	8	34,8

The mean duration of disease in patients with Crohn's disease was estimated at 3.50 ± 3.29 years.

5.1.5.2. Haemorrhagic rectocolitis (UC)

Of our 57 patients with UC, 27 (47.4%) were anaemic.

Recto-sigmoid location was the most common (46.4%), followed by pan-colonic location (30.4%) (Table III).

More than half of these patients (52.6%) presented with an inaugural flare-up deemed minimal according to the Montreal classification, compared with 46.2% who presented with a severe inaugural flare-up. The latter patients all had anaemia.

The mean duration of UC in our patients was 8.33±5 years.

Table IIIV: Distribution of UC patients according to the extent of their disease (Montreal classification)

Montreal classification	*Non-anaemic group % (n=30)*	*Anaemic group % (n=27)*
E1: Rectitis	47,5	15,0
E2: Left colitis	17,5	17,5
E3: Pancolic	7,5	35,0

5.1.6. Clinical data

The clinical signs most frequently found during the inaugural outbreak were dominated by glairosanguineous diarrhoea in both anaemic and non-anaemic patients (Table IV).

Table IV: Breakdown of patients by main clinical group occurring during inaugural attacks

	Group of anaemic patients (N=40)		*Group of non-anaemic patients (N=40)*	
	Number of patients	*%*	*Number of patients*	*%*
Presence of glairosanguineous diarrhoea	34	85	33	82,5
Presence of watery diarrhoea	6	15	3	7,5
Presence of subocclusive syndrome	5	12,5	1	2,5
Presence of abdominal pain	25	62,5	15	37,5

All non-anaemic patients had an estimated WHO score of 0. For anaemic patients, 7 (17.9%) patients had an estimated score of 1, 2 patients (5.1%) had an estimated score of 2 and only 1 patient (2.6%) had an estimated score of score of 3. The remaining anaemic patients (74.4%) had a score of 0. The anaemic patients had a higher mean heart rate than our non-anaemic patients: 86.84 ± 8.64 beats/min VS 76.85 ± 18.4 beats/min.

Of the ten patients with extradigestive manifestations of IBD, five had sacroiliitis, two had osteopenia and one had uveitis.

The mean BMI was 24.07 kg/m^2 and 21.77 kg/m^2 for non-anaemic and anaemic patients respectively. Among our anaemic patients, 11 had a BMI < 18.5 kg/m 2 (27.5%), 9 were overweight (22.5%), only 1 patient was obese (2.5%) and the others had a normal body mass (47.5%).

However, among our non-anaemic patients, 6 had a BMI < 18.5 kg/m^2 (15%), 20 were overweight (50%), 1 was obese (2.5%) and the remainder had a normal body index (32.5%).

Among the anaemic patients, 39 had had an examination of the anal margin, of whom 33 (84.6%) had a normal examination, 5.1% had fistulas and 10.3% had fissures.

Of the patients without anaemia, 39 had an anal margin examination, of whom 92.3% had a normal examination, 5.1% had fistulas and 2.6% had fissures (Table V).

Table VI: Distribution of patients according to proctological examination data

		Non-anaemic patients		*Anaemic patients*	
		N=39	*%*	*N=39*	*%*
Examination of the anal margin	Normal	36	92,3	33	84,6
	Fistulas	2	5,1	2	5,1
	Cracks	1	2,6	4	10,3

5.1.7. Biological data

5.1.7.1. Characteristics of anaemia

In the majority of our anaemic patients, 29 (72.5%), the anaemia was discovered during the inaugural attack.

The mean haemoglobin value was 13.83 g/l in non-anaemic patients compared with 10.39 g/l in patients in the anaemic group (Table VII).

In the case of anaemic patients, 96% of those with an elevated CRP (greater than 6) had advanced disease and 92% were hospitalised.

Table VII: Distribution of patients according to biological data

	Without anaemia		*With anaemia*	
	Average	***Standard deviation***	***Average***	***Standard deviation***
Hb (in g/l)	13,83	1,068	10,39	1,69
VGM (in FL)	86,30	5,10	78,15	8,83
Ht (%)	41,12	3,08	32,37	4,54
WBC (E /mm3)	6559,05	2020,15	9774,73	7258,95
Plt(E /mm3)	271475	89048,24	331175	110487,47
CRP (mg/l)	13,04	17,60	35,36	49,89
SV at 1st hour in min	19,38	16,03	40,75	28,27
Ferritinemia (ug/l)	43,42	27,45	70,61	122,38

Hb: haemoglobin; WBC: white blood cells; VGM: mean corpuscular volume; CRP: C-reactive protein; VS: sedimentation rate; Plt: platelets; HT: haematocrit.

Anemia was microcytic in more than half the patients and no cases of macrocytic anemia were observed (Figure 1).

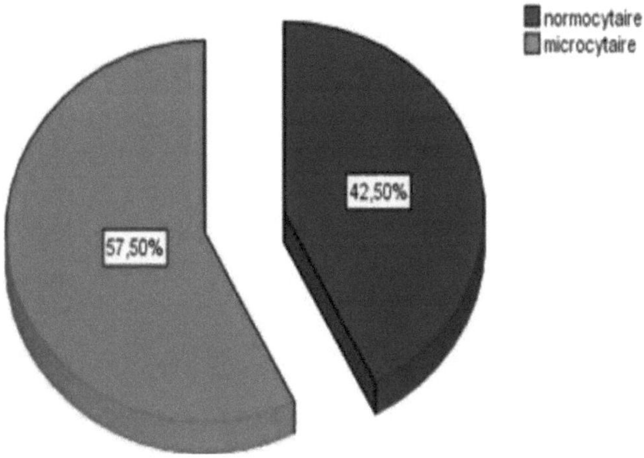

Figure 1:* *Distribution of patients according to type of anaemia

Taking into account the data of the martial and inflammatory assessment, we retained :

- A martial deficiency was the predominant cause of anaemia in 20 patients (50%).
- Inflammatory anaemia was the predominant cause in 7 patients (17.5%).
- A mixed cause of anaemia (deficiency and inflammatory) in 13 patients (32.5%).

These results are illustrated in Figure 2.

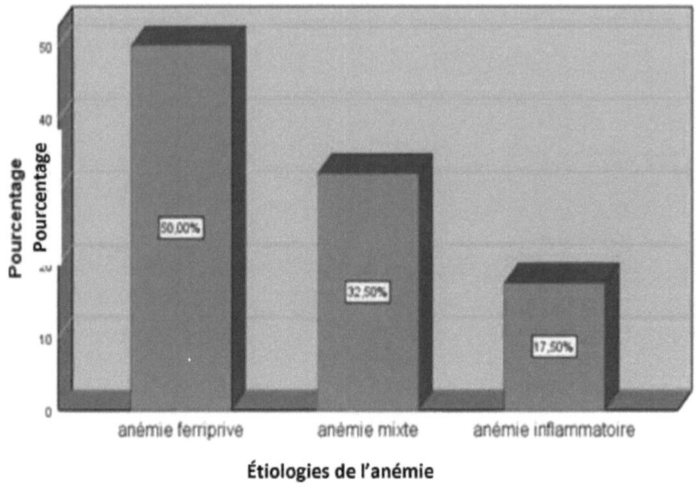

Figure 2: Main causes of anaemia in our IBD patients

Vitamin B12 deficiency was found in 4 (14.3%) of the 28 patients who had vitamin B12 levels measured, including only one patient with Crohn's disease.

Folate deficiency was found in 10 anaemic patients (37.5%) out of 28 patients who had a folate assay, including three with Crohn's disease.

None of our anaemic patients had had an LDH, haptoglobin, reticulocyte or direct Coombs test at the onset of their anaemia.

5.1.7.2. Nutritional assessment

Hypo albuminemia was present in 34 patients (42.5%). Most of these patients were anaemic (60%). Hypocalcaemia was present in 14 patients (17.5%), 8 of whom were anaemic and 6 non-anaemic. Hypomagnesaemia was present in 5 patients (6.3%), 4 of whom were anaemic and 1 non-anaemic.

Hypocholesterolaemia was present in 11 patients (13.75%), 7 of whom were anaemic and 4 non-anaemic. Hypotriglyceridaemia was present in 7 patients (8.8%), 5 of whom were anaemic and 2 non-anaemic.

5.1.7.2. Other biological data

Renal function was impaired in only one patient. He had anaemia. Hypokalaemia was present in 8 patients (10%), the majority of whom were anaemic (87.5%).

Hyponatremia was present in 3 patients (3.8%), all of whom were anaemic.

Hepatocellular function was normal in all our patients.

Serum pANCA levels were positive in 9 patients (11.3%), 5 anaemic and 4 non-anaemic.

Serum ASCA levels were positive in 2 patients, including one with anaemia.

A total of 26 patients (32.5%) had hypergammaglobulinaemia, 17 of whom were anaemic and 9 non-anaemic. Three patients (3.8%) had hypogammaglobulinaemia, including two anaemic patients.

Among our patients, 35 (43.8%) had a blood ferritin level below 30 pg/l and 10 (12.5%) had a blood ferritin level above 100pg/l. In addition, 21 (52.1%) anaemic patients had a martial deficiency compared with 15 non-anaemic patients (37.5%).

5.1.7.3. Endoscopic data

All our anaemic patients underwent colonoscopy at the onset of their anaemia, 77.5% of whom had active disease.

Of our patients, 48 (60%) underwent fibroscopy at the initial diagnosis of the disease and 26 patients at the onset of anaemia. This examination revealed loss of gastric, duodenal and/or bulbar substances in 4 patients (8.3%), 3 of whom (7.6%) were anaemic.

A duodenal mosaic appearance was found in a single anaemic patient.

Pathological examination showed that 32 patients (66.6%) had an Hp infection, 15 (44.11%) of whom were anaemic. Duodenal atrophy was present in 4 patients, 3 of whom were anaemic (Table VIII).

Table VIII: Distribution of patients according to endoscopic and anatomopathological data from oesogastroduodenal fibroscopy

		Without anaemia		*With anaemia*	
		Number (n=22)	***%***	***Number (n=26)***	***%***
Gastric endoscopic data	Ulceration	1	2,5	1	2,5
	Nodules	2	5	5	12,5
	Erosion	1	2,5	2	5
	Normal	15	37,5	17	42,5
Duodenal endoscopic data	Erosion	1	2,5	1	2,5
	Mosaic	0	0	1	2,5
	Normal	18	45	21	52,5
Bulbar endoscopic data	Ulceration	0	0	2	5
	Normal	18	45	21	52,5
Results of anatomopathological examination of biopsies	Gastric Atrophy	6	15	11	27,5
	Gastric metaplasia	0	0	1	2,5
	Hp	17	42,5	15	37,5
	Duodenal atrophy	1	2,5	3	7,5

5.1.7.4. Therapeutic features

Treatment of IBD flare-ups:

Regarding the treatments received at the time of the flare-ups, we found significantly more patients on corticosteroids (systemic route) in the anaemic group (62.5%) than in the non-anaemic group (37.5%) (p =0.025).

Maintenance treatment:

Among the anaemic patients, 52.5% received immunosuppressive treatment, compared with 12.5% of non-anaemic patients. Only one patient was treated with methotrexate. This treatment was discontinued 2 months after the onset of his anaemia. All the others were on azathiorpine.

Only one anaemic patient was put on anti TNF a. He had Crohn's disease. Treatment was discontinued 3 years after the onset of anaemia. He had recurrent anaemia.

Compliance with treatment:

Among 39 anaemic patients, 7 (17.9%) had poor compliance with their treatment. Only one anaemic patient was not compliant.

Of the 40 non-anaemic patients, 7 (17.5%) had poor compliance.

Undesirable effects of treatment:

Among the 40 non-anaemic patients, 7 (17.5%) had adverse reactions to maintenance treatment. These included dyspnoea, epigastralgia, skin rash and pruritus. In contrast, 4 (10%) patients in the group of anaemic patients had signs of drug intolerance. These included epigastralgia, rash and peripheral polyneuropathy. Only one anaemic patient presented with neutropenia, after 10 months from the onset of the anaemia, the other blood lines were not affected (Table IX).

Table IX: Undesirable effects of treatments in our population

	With anaemia		*Without anaemia*	
	Number n=4	*%*	*Number n=7*	*%*
Epigastralgia	1	25	1	14,3
Skin rash	1	25	3	42,9
Pruritus			2	28,6
Dyspnoea			1	14,3
Neutropenia	1	25		
Polyneuropathy	1	25		

Treatment of ¡anaemia:

Of our anaemic patients, 28 (70%) received treatment for their anaemia.

Of the patients who received treatment for their anaemia, 17.9% received a blood transfusion, 96.4% received oral supplementation and only 21.4% received intravenous ferric hydroxide-sucrose (Veinofer®) martial therapy. The patients who received a blood transfusion all had haemoglobin levels below 8.5g/l.

Of the twelve patients who had not received martial therapy or transfusion, 8 had improved anaemia.

Progressive features of anaemia :

The course of the anaemia was marked by its disappearance in 45% of cases, its persistence in 42.5% of cases and its recurrence in 12.5% of cases.

5.2. Analytical study

5.2.1. Uni-varied study

5.2.1.1. Comparison of the 2 groups according to epidemiological data

There were no statistically significant differences between the two groups in terms of age, sex, family history of IBD or lifestyle habits (Table X).

Table X: Comparison of the two groups according to epidemiological characteristics

	Anaemic group	*Non-anaemic group*	*p*
Average age (years)	50,62	45,42	0.122
Female (%)	65	45	0,072
Smokers (%)	20	17,5	0,775
Alcohol consumers (%)	7,5	2,5	0,305
Family history of IBD (%)	12,5	0	0,055
Long-term PPI treatment (%)	12,5	20	0,363

IBD: inflammatory bowel disease; PPI: proton pump inhibitors.

Similarly, there was no statistically significant difference in the type of IBD between the group of anaemic and non-anaemic patients (Table XI).

Table VIIII: Comparison of our patients according to IBD type

		Without anaemia	*With anaemia*	*P*
Type of IBD	UC (N=57)	52,6	47,4	0,459
	Crohn's (N=23)	43,5	56,5	

IBD: inflammatory bowel disease; UC: haemorrhagic rectocolitis

5.2.1.2. Comparison of the 2 groups according to the characteristics of Crohn's disease

Anaemic patients with Crohn's disease had a longer duration of disease than non-anaemic patients, with a statistically significant difference between the two groups (4.79 ± 3.4 years Vs 1.81 ± 2.33 years, p=0.027). Similarly, anaemic patients were hospitalised more frequently than non-anaemic patients (p=0.000).

In the group of anaemic patients with Crohn's disease, the location and severity of the first attack and the mode of progression were not associated with the presence of anaemia (Table XII).

Table IXII: Comparison of the two groups according to disease characteristics in patients with Crohn's disease

		Anaemic	*Non anaemic*	*P*
Age at diagnosis (%)	A1	61,5	60	1
	A2	61,5	60	1
	A3	23,1	30	1
Location (%)	L1	23,1	40	0,650
	L2	7,7	10	1
	L3	69,2	50	0,417
	L4	0	0	0,650
Evolutionary mode (%)	B1	69,2	80	
	B2	15,4	10	1
	B3	15,4	10	1
Perineal damage (%)	P	15,4	20	1
Severity of the inaugural attack (according to the CDAI index)	Minimal activity (%)	7,7	20	0,103
	Moderate activity (%)	38,5	70	
	Severe activity (%)	53,8	10	
Average duration of disease (in years)		4,79	1,81	**0,027**
Total number of hospitalisations (%)	0	15,4	70	**0,026**
	1	69,2	30	
	2	15,4	0	
Total number of attacks (%)	0	15,4	10	0,604
	1	69,2	90	
	2	15,4	0	
Number of severe attacks (%)	0	92,3	100	1
	1	7,7	0	

CDAI: Crohn's disease activity index or CD activity score

5.2.1.3. Comparison of the 2 groups according to UC characteristics.

For UC, pan-colonic localisation was found in 52% of anaemic patients compared with only 10% of non-anaemic patients, with a significant difference between the two groups (p=0.001). On the other hand, recto-sigmoid localisation was more frequently found in non-anaemic patients with a statistically significant difference (63.3% Vs 22.2%; p=0.002). In addition, there was a significant difference between the two groups in terms of the severity of the inaugural attack (p<0.0001).

Patients with anaemia were more frequently hospitalised and had more relapses and severe relapses, with statistically significant differences of p<0.0001, p<0.0001 and p<0.0001 respectively.

The mean duration of UC in the non-anaemic group was 9.69 ± 6.69 years, compared with 6.81 ± 4.56 years in the anaemic group, but the difference was not significant (p=0.061) (Table XIII).

Table XII: Comparison of the two groups according to disease characteristics in patients with UC

		Group 1 (Anaemic)	*Group 2 (No anaemia)*	*p*
Location (%)	E1	22,2	63,3	**0,002**
	E2	25,9	23,3	0,820
	E3	51,9	10	**0,001**
Severity of inaugural attack (according to Montréal classification) (%)	S1	38,5	70	**0,000**
	S2	15,4	30	
	S3	46,2		
Average duration of disease (years)		6,81	9,69	0,061
	0	22,2	83,3	**0,000**

Total number of hospitalisations (%)	1	63	16,7	
		11,1	0	
		3,7	0	
Total number of pushes (%)		3,7	3,3	0,703
		44,4	50	
		29,6	36,7	
		22,2	10	
Number of severe attacks (%)		55,6	96,7	**0,000**
		44,4	3,3	

5.2.1.4. Comparison of the 2 groups according to clinical data at the time of the first attack

Among our anaemic patients, 65% presented with abdominal pain Vs 37.5% with a statistically significant difference (p=0.014). In addition, all non-anaemic patients had an estimated WHO score of 0 compared with 74.4% of anaemic patients, with a statistically significant difference (p=0.01). Furthermore, anaemic patients had a higher mean heart rate than our non-anaemic patients with a statistically significant difference (p=0.013).

In the group of patients without anaemia, overweight was more frequent (50% Vs 22.5%) with a statistically significant difference (p=0.011) (Table XIV).

Table XIV: Comparison of the two groups according to clinical data at the time of the inaugural attack

<table>
<tr><th colspan="2"></th><th>Anaemic</th><th>Non anaemic</th><th>P</th></tr>
<tr><td rowspan="4">Symptoms during inaugural attacks (%)</td><td>Glaucous diarrhoea</td><td>72,5</td><td>82,5</td><td>0,284</td></tr>
<tr><td>Watery diarrhoea</td><td>17,5</td><td>7,5</td><td>0,311</td></tr>
<tr><td>Subocclusive syndrome</td><td>10</td><td>2,5</td><td>0,359</td></tr>
<tr><td>Abdominal pain</td><td>65</td><td>37,5</td><td>0,014</td></tr>
<tr><td rowspan="2">WHO score (%)</td><td>0</td><td>74,4</td><td>100</td><td rowspan="2">0,001</td></tr>
<tr><td>> 0</td><td>25,6</td><td>0</td></tr>
<tr><td colspan="2">Average heart rate (beats/min)</td><td>86,82</td><td>76,85</td><td>0,003</td></tr>
<tr><td colspan="2">Non-digestive symptoms (%)</td><td>10</td><td>10</td><td>1</td></tr>
<tr><td rowspan="4">Body mass index (%)</td><td>Slim</td><td>27,5</td><td>15</td><td>0,172</td></tr>
<tr><td>Normal</td><td>47,5</td><td>32,5</td><td>0,171</td></tr>
<tr><td>Overweight</td><td>22,5</td><td>50</td><td>0,011</td></tr>
<tr><td>Obese</td><td>2,5</td><td>2,5</td><td>1</td></tr>
<tr><td rowspan="3">Proctological examination (%)</td><td>Cracks</td><td>10</td><td>2,5</td><td>0,359</td></tr>
<tr><td>Fistulas</td><td>5</td><td>5</td><td>1</td></tr>
<tr><td>Normal</td><td>82,5</td><td>90</td><td>0,518</td></tr>
</table>

WHO: World Health Organization

5.2.1.5. Comparison of the 2 groups according to biological data

As expected, the mean haemoglobin value was higher in the non-anaemic group (13.83 g/l vs 10.3 g/l) with a statistically significant difference ($p=0.000$). Similarly, mean haematocrit and mean corpuscular volume were significantly lower in anaemic patients, with $p<0.0001$ and $p<0.0001$ respectively. In contrast, mean white blood cell and platelet counts were significantly higher in anaemic patients compared with non-anaemic patients ($p=0.01$; $p=0.009$ respectively). However, mean ferritin levels were not significantly different between the two groups (43.42 pg/l vs 70.62 pg/l ; p=0.183), unlike mean SV and CRP levels, which were significantly higher in anaemic patients compared with non-anaemic patients (respectively 40.75± 28.27 Vs 19.3 8± 16.03; p<0.0001 and 35.36± 49.89 mg/l Vs 13.04± 17.60 mg/l; p<0.001) (Table XV).

Table XV: Comparison of the 2 groups according to the results of the haemogram and inflammatory assessment

		Without anaemia	*With anaemia*	*P*
Hb in g/l		13,83	10,38	**0,000**
VGM in FL		86,31	78,15	**0,000**
Ht in		41,12	32,37	**0,000**
Gb (E/mm^3)		6559	9774,7	**0,010**
Plt (E/mm^3)		271475	331175	**0,009**
CRP (mg/l)		13,04	35,36	**0,010**
SV at 1ère hour (min)		19,37	40,75	**0,000**
Ferritinemia (gg/D	Average value	43,42	27,45	0,183
	< 30pg/l as%.	18,8	25	0,260
	> 100pg/l as a	3,8	8,8	0,311

Hb: serum haemoglobin level; WBC: white blood cells; mean corpuscular volume; CRP: C-reactive protein; SV: sedimentation rate; PLT: platelets; HT: haematocrit

With regard to other biological parameters, hypoalbuminemia was more frequent in anaemic patients, with a statistically significant difference (p=0.002).

With regard to ionic disorders, serum creatinine and urea levels, there was no significant difference between the two groups (Table XVI).

Table XIII: Comparison of the 2 groups according to biological data

	Anaemic	*Non anaemic*	*p*
Hypokalaemia (%)	17,5	2,7	0,057
Hyponatremia (%)	7,5		0,241
Renal insufficiency (%)	2,5		1
ASCA (+) (%)	2,5	2,5	1
ANCA (+) (%)	10	12,5	1
Hypo albuminemia (%)	60	25	**0,002**
Hypergammaglobulinemia (%)	57,5	22,5	0,056
Hypogammaglobulinemia (%)	5	2,5	1
Hypocalcaemia (corrected)(%)	20	15	0,556
Hypomagnesaemia (%)	10	2,5	0,359
Hypocholesterolaemia (%)	17,5	10	0,518
Hypotriglyceridaemia (%)	12,5	5	0,432

ASCA: Anti-Saccharomyces cerevisiae antibody; ANCA: Anti-neutrophil cytoplasmic autoantibody

5.2.1.6. Comparison of the 2 groups according to endoscopic and anatomopathological data

With regard to endoscopic and anatomopathological parameters, we found no significant difference between the two groups (Table XVII).

Table XIIIII: Comparison of the 2 groups according to the data endoscopic and anatomopathological

		No anaemia n=22		*With anaemia n=26*		***P***
		Frequency	***%***	***Frequency***	***%***	
Gastric endoscopic data	Ulceration	1	2,5	1	2,5	1
	Nodules	2	5	5	12,5	0,432
	Erosion	1	2,5	2	5	1
	Normal	15	37,5	17	42,5	0,648
Duodenal endoscopic data	Ulceration	0	0	0	0	
	Nodules	0	0	0	0	
	Erosion	1	2,5	1	2,5	1
	Mosaic	0	0	1	2,5	1
	Normal	18	45	21	52,5	0,370
Bulbar endoscopic data	Ulceration	0	0	2	5	0,494
	Normal	18	45	21	52,5	0,502
Results of anatomopathological examination s of biopsies	Gastric atrophy	6	15	11	27,5	0,172
	Gastric metaplasia	0	0	1	2,5	1
	Hp	17	42,5	15	37,5	0,648
	Duodenal atrophy	1	2,5	3	7,5	0,615

Hp: Helicobacter pylori

5.2.1.7. Comparison of the 2 groups according to therapeutic characteristics

In terms of treatment modalities, systemic corticosteroids were used more frequently in the anaemic group, with a statistically significant difference ($p=0.025$). Similarly, 52.5% of anaemic patients received immunosuppressive treatment compared with 12.5% of non-anaemic patients, with a statistically significant difference ($p<0.0001$). However, there was no significant difference between the two groups in terms of compliance with treatment or the frequency of adverse drug reactions (Table XVIII).

Table XIVII: Comparison of the two groups according to therapeutic characteristics

	Anaemic group	*Non-anaemic group*	*p*
Use of systemic corticosteroids (%)	62,5	37,5	**0,025**
Use of immunosuppressants (%)	52,5	12,5	**0,000**
Poor compliance with medication (%)	17,5	17,5	1
Undesirable effects of treatments (%)	10	17,5	0,518

5.2.2. Multi-variety study

The factors retained as independent factors associated with anaemia in IBD were (Table XIX) :

- BMI<25kg/m^2 : OR =3 (CI = [0.99-9.04], p=0.051).
- Female: OR=2.605 (CI [0.908-7.470], p =0.075).
- Hypoalbuminemia: OR=4.273 (CI [1.467-12.449], p =0.008).

- Heart rate: If heart rate increases, the risk of developing anaemia is multiplied by 5.2% with an estimated threshold of 87 beats/min OR=1.05 (CI [1.00-1.10], p =0.023).

Table XVX: Multivariate study looking for independent factors in the occurrence of anaemia in IBD

			95% confidence interval	
	P	***Exp(B)***	***Lower***	***Superior***
Hypoalbuminemia	0,008	4,273	1,467	12,449
Heart rate	0,023	1,052	1,007	1,100
Female sex	0,075	2,605	0,908	7,470
BMI< 25kg/m^2	0,051	3,000	0,995	9,045

BMI: body mass index

5.2.3. Factors associated with persistence and/or recurrence of anaemia

We compared the demographic, clinical, endoscopic and biological characteristics of anaemic patients according to the course of the anaemia. We considered two groups of patients, the first comprising those whose anaemia had disappeared (group A, N=18 patients) and the second including those whose anaemia had either persisted or recurred (N=22 patients, group B).

Patients with persistent/recurrent anaemia had a significantly lower mean age (41.04 ± 14.67 years VS 50.77 ± 10.81 years respectively, **p=0.025**) and a lower initial haemoglobin level (9.83g/l ± 1.88 Vs 11.06g/l ±1.14; **p=0.016)** (Table XIX).

With regard to clinical signs, patients with persistent and/or recurrent anaemia had more glairo-bloody diarrhoea at the time of the inagural attack than patients with improved anaemia (86.4% versus 55.6% with **p=0.04**). There was no significant difference between the two groups with regard to sex, BMI value and other clinical, biological, endoscopic, anatomopathological and therapeutic parameters (Tables XX, XXI, XXII, XXIII, XXIV, XXV, XXVI and XXVII).

Table XX: Comparison of the two groups according to epidemiological data

	Group A	*Group B*	*P*
Average age (years)	50,77	41,04	**0,025**
Female (%)	50	77,3	0,072
Smokers (%)	27,8	13,6	0,430
Alcohol consumers (%)	11,1	4,5	0,579
Family history of IBD (%)	11,1	13,6	1

ATCD: antecedents, IBD: inflammatory bowel disease

<u>Table XVII:</u> Comparison of the two groups according to disease characteristics in patients with Crohn's disease

<table>
<tr><th colspan="2"></th><th>Group A</th><th>Group B</th><th>P</th></tr>
<tr><td rowspan="3">Age at diagnosis</td><td>A1 (%)</td><td>14,3</td><td>16,7</td><td>1</td></tr>
<tr><td>A2 (%)</td><td>42,9</td><td>83,3</td><td>0,266</td></tr>
<tr><td>A3 (%)</td><td>42,9</td><td>0</td><td>0,192</td></tr>
<tr><td rowspan="3">Location</td><td>L1 (%)</td><td>14,3</td><td>33,3</td><td>0,559</td></tr>
<tr><td>L2 (%)</td><td>14,3</td><td>0</td><td>1</td></tr>
<tr><td>L3 (%)</td><td>71,4</td><td>66,7</td><td>1</td></tr>
<tr><td rowspan="3">Scalable mode</td><td>B1 (%)</td><td>85,7</td><td>50</td><td>0,266</td></tr>
<tr><td>B2 (%)</td><td>14,3</td><td>16,7</td><td>1</td></tr>
<tr><td>B3 (%)</td><td>0</td><td>33,3</td><td>0,192</td></tr>
<tr><td colspan="2">Perineal damage p (%)</td><td>14,3</td><td>16,7</td><td>1</td></tr>
<tr><td rowspan="3">Severity of inaugural attack (according to CDAI index)</td><td>Not active (%)</td><td>0</td><td>16,7</td><td rowspan="3">1</td></tr>
<tr><td>Minimal activity (%)</td><td>42,9</td><td>33,3</td></tr>
<tr><td>Moderate activity (%)</td><td>57,1</td><td>50</td></tr>
<tr><td rowspan="3">Total number of hospitalisations (%)</td><td>0</td><td>28,6</td><td>0</td><td rowspan="3">0,706</td></tr>
<tr><td>1</td><td>57,1</td><td>83,3</td></tr>
<tr><td>2</td><td>14,3</td><td>16,7</td></tr>
<tr><td rowspan="3">Total number of attacks (%)</td><td>0</td><td>14,3</td><td>16,7</td><td rowspan="3">1</td></tr>
<tr><td>1</td><td>71,4</td><td>66,7</td></tr>
<tr><td>2</td><td>14,3</td><td>16,7</td></tr>
<tr><td rowspan="2">Number of severe attacks (%)</td><td>0</td><td>0</td><td>83,3</td><td rowspan="2">0,462</td></tr>
<tr><td>1</td><td>0</td><td>16,7</td></tr>
</table>

CDAI: Crohn's disease activity index or CD activity score

Table XVIIII: Comparison of disease characteristics in patients with UC between group A and group B

		Group A	*Group B*	*P*
Location (%)	El	27,3	18,8	0,662
	E2	27,3	25	1
	E3	45,5	56,3	0,704
Severity of onset (according to Montéral classification) (%)	S1	45,5	33,3	0,667
	S2	18,2	13,3	
	S3	36,4	53,3	
Total number of hospitalisations (%)	0	27,3	18,8	0,692
	1	54,5	68,8	
	2	9,1	12,5	
	3	9,1		
Total number of pushes (%)	0	54,5	6,3	0,622
	1	18,2	37,5	
	2	27,3	37,5	
	3	0	18,8	
Number of severe attacks (%)	0	63,6	50	0,696
	1	36,4	50	

Table XVIIIII: Comparison of the two groups according to clinical data at the inaugural attack

		Group A	*Group B*	*P*
Symptoms during inaugural attacks (%)	Glaucous diarrhoea	55,6	86,4	**0,04**
	Watery diarrhoea	16,7	18,2	1
	Subocclusive syndrome	5,6	13,6	0,613
	Abdominal pain	55,6	72,7	0,257
WHO score (%)	0	82,4	68,2	0,082
	> 0	17,7	31,8	
Average heart rate (beats/min)		85,33	88,04	0,649
Non-digestive symptoms (%)		11,1	9,1	1
Body mass index (%)	Slim	16,7	36,4	0,286
	Normal	61,1	36,4	0,119
	Overweight	22,2	22,7	1
	Obese	0	4,5	1
Proctological examination (%)	Cracks	11,11	9,1	1
	Fistulas	5,6	4,5	1
	Normal	77,8	86,4	0,680

WHO: World Health Organization

Table XIXV: Comparison of the 2 groups according to the results of the haemogram and inflammatory assessment

	Group A	*Group B*	*P*
Hbt (g/l)	11,05	9,84	**0,016**
VGM (FL)	77,92	78,34	0,885
Ht (%)	34,82	30,37	0,001
Gb (E/mm^3)	8408	10892	0,287
Plt (E/mm^3)	305444	352227	0,186
Crp (mg/l)	34,03	36,45	0,881
SV at 1st hour (min)	34,44	45,90	0,206
Average value	58,99	79,60	0,608
Ferritinemia (pg/l) 30 pg/l <(%)	22,5	27,5	1
> 100 pg/l (%)	7,5	10,0	1

Hb: serum haemoglobin level; WBC: white blood cells; mean corpuscular volume; CRP: C-reactive protein; SV: sedimentation rate; PLT: platelets; HT: haematocrit.

Table XX: Comparison of the two groups according to other biological parameters

	Group A	*Group B*	*p*
Hypokalaemia (%)	11,1	22,7	0,427
Hyponatremia (%)	5	9,1	1
Renal insufficiency (%)	5,6	0	0,45
ASCA (in %)	5,6	0	0,45
ANCA (in %)	11,1	9,1	0,617
Hypo albuminemia (in %)	66	54,5	0,436
Hypergammaglobulinaemia (%)	33,3	50	0,348
Hypogammaglobulinemia (%)	5,6	4,5	1
Hypocalcaemia (corrected) (%)	11,1	27,3	0,258
Hypomagnesaemia (%)	5,6	13,6	0,613
Hypocholesterolaemia (%)	16,7	18,2	1
Hypotriglyceridaemia (%)	16,7	9,1	0,642

ASCA: Anti-Saccharomyces cerevisiae antibody; ANCA: Anti-neutrophil cytoplasmic autoantibody

Table XXII: Comparison of endoscopic and anatomopathological parameters between group A and group B

		Group A		*Group B*		*P*
		Frequency	*As a % of*	*Frequency*	*As a % of*	
Gastric endoscopic data	Ulceration	0	0	1	4,5	1
	Nodules	1	5,6	4	18,2	0,355
	Erosion	1	5,6	1	4,5	1
	Normal	9	50	8	36,4	0,385
Duodenal endoscopic	Erosion	0	0	1	4,5	1

data	Mosaic	0		1	4,5	1
	Normal	10	55,6	11	50	0,726
Bulbar endoscopic data	Ulceration	1	5,6	1	4,5	1
	Normal	9	50	12	54,5	0,775
Results of anatomopathological examination of biopsies	Gastric Atrophy	4	2,2	7	31,8	0,723
	Gastric metaplasia	1	5,6	0	0	0,450
	Hp	7	38,9	8	36,4	0,870
	Duodenal atrophy	0	0%	3	13,6	0,238

Hp: Helicobacter pylori

Table XXIIII: Comparison of therapeutic characteristics between Group A and Group B

	Group A	*Group B*	*P*
Use of systemic corticosteroids (%)	61,1	63,6	0,870
Use of immunosuppressants (%)	11,1	9,1	1
Poor compliance (%)	16,7	18,2	1
Undesirable effects of treatments (%)	44,4	59,1	0,356

CHAPTER VI. OUTLOOK

A prospective study with a sufficiently long follow-up of a sufficient number of patients and a study of all the parameters involved in the pathogenesis of anaemia would enable a more in-depth analysis of the association between anaemia and IBD.

REFERENCES

1. Kuznicki P, Neubauer K. Emerging comorbidities in inflammatory bowel disease: Eating disorders, alcohol and narcotics misuse. J Clin Med. 2021;10(19).

2. Tulewicz-marti E, Moniuszko A, Rydzewska G. Management of anemia in inflammatory bowel disease: a challenge in everyday clinical practice. Gastroenterol Rev. 2017;12(4):239-243.

3. Mahadea D, Adamczewska E, Rataj czak AE, Rychter AM, Zawada A, Eder P, et al. Iron deficiency anemia in inflammatory bowel diseases-a narrative review. Nutrients. 2021;13(11).

4. Gargallo-Puyuelo CJ, Alfambra E, García-Erce JA, Gomollon F. Iron treatment may be difficult in inflammatory diseases: Inflammatory bowel disease as a paradigm. Nutrients. 2018;10(12):1-14.

5. Aksan A, Beales ILP, Baxter G, de Arellano AR, Gavata S, Valentine WJ, et al. Evaluation of the cost-effectiveness of iron formulations for the treatment of iron deficiency in patients with inflammatory bowel disease in the UK. Clin Outcomes Res. 2021;13(June):541-52.

6. Göksel Bengi, Hatice Keyvan, Seda Bayrak Durmaz HA. Frequency, types, and treatment of anemia in Turkish patients with inflammatory bowel disease. World J Gastroenterol. 2018;24(36):4186-96.

7. Resál T, Farkas K, Molnár T. Iron Deficiency Anemia in Inflammatory Bowel Disease: What Do We Know? Front Med. 2021;8(July).

8. Akhuemonkhan E, Parian A, Miller K, Hanauer S, Hutfless S. Prevalence and screening for anaemia in mild to moderate Crohn's disease and

ulcerative colitis in the United States, 2010-2014. BMJ Open Gastroenterol. 2017;4(1):1-8.

9. Foteinogiannopoulou K, Karmiris K, Axiaris G, Velegraki M, Gklavas A, Kapizioni C, et al. The burden and management of anemia in Greek patients with inflammatory bowel disease: a retrospective, multicenter, observational study. BMC Gastroenterol [Internet]. 2021;21(1):1-10. Available from: https://doi.org/10.1186/s12876-021-01826-1

10. Antunes CVDA, Hallack Neto AE, Nascimento CRDA, Chebli LA, Moutinho ILD, Pinheiro BDV, et al. Anemia in inflammatory bowel disease outpatients: Prevalence, risk factors, and etiology. Biomed Res Int. 2015;2015.

11. Maaser C, Sturm A, Vavricka SR, Kucharzik T, Fiorino G, Annese V, et al. ECCO Guideline / Consensus Paper ECCO-ESGAR Guideline for Diagnostic Assessment in IBD Part 1 : Initial diagnosis , monitoring of known IBD , detection of complications. J Crohn's Colitis. 2019;144-64.

12. Mak WY, Zhao M, Ng SC, Burisch J. The epidemiology of inflammatory bowel disease: east meets west. J Gastroenterol Hepatol. 2020;35(3):380- 9.

13. Schoepfer AM, Beglinger C, Straumann A, Safroneeva E, Romero Y, Armstrong D, et al. Fecal calprotectin more accurately reflects endoscopic activity of ulcerative colitis than the lichtiger index, C-reactive protein, platelets, hemoglobin, and blood leukocytes. Inflamm Bowel Dis. 2013;19(2):332-41.

14. Ochsenkühn T, Tillack C, Szokodi D, Janelidze S, Schnitzler F. Clinical outcomes with ustekinumab as rescue treatment in therapy-refractory or therapy-intolerant ulcerative colitis. United Eur Gastroenterol J.

2020;8(1):91-8.

15. WHO. Haemoglobin concentrations used to diagnose anaemia and assess its severity. Nutr information system vitamins minerals [Internet]. 2011;1-6. Available from: http://www.who.int/vmnis/indicators/haemoglobin_ en.pdfl -6

16. Lamb CA, Kennedy NA, Raine T, Hendy PA, Smith PJ, Limdi JK, et al. British Society of Gastroenterology consensus guidelines on the management of inflammatory bowel disease in adults. Gut. 2019;68:s1- 106.

17. Gisbert JP, Gomollón F. Common misconceptions in the diagnosis and management of anemia in inflammatory bowel disease. Am J Gastroenterol. 2008;103(5):1299-307.

18. Filmann N, Math D, Rey J, Math D, Schneeweiss S, Ardizzone S, et al. Prevalence of Anemia in In fl ammatory Bowel Diseases in European Countries: A Systematic Review and Individual Patient Data. Inflamm Bowel Dis. 2014;20(5).

19. 1 MW, , Anna Borkowska 2 and Renata Talar-Wojnarowska 1,* , Marta Jastrz^ebska 3, Marcin Sochal 4 EM-W 1, 1. Clinical and Laboratory Characteristics of Anaemia in Hospitalized Patients with Inflammatory Bowel Disease. J Clin Med Artic. 2023;

20. Kaitha S, Bashir M, Ali T. Iron deficiency anemia in inflammatory bowel disease. World J Gastrointest Pathophysiol. 2015;6(3):62.

21. Stein J, Hartmann F, Dignass AU. Diagnosis and management of iron deficiency anemia in patients with IBD. Nat Rev Gastroenterol Hepatol [Internet]. 2010;7(11):599-610. Available

Available from:

http : //dx.doi. org/10.1038/nrgastro .2010.151

22. Dignass AU, Gasche C, Bettenworth D, Birgegârd G, Danese S, Gisbert JP, et al. European consensus on the diagnosis and management of iron deficiency and anaemia in inflammatory bowel diseases. J Crohn's Colitis. 2015;9(3):211-22.

23. Ioannis E. Koutroubakis, MD, Claudia Ramos-Rivers, MD, Miguel Regueiro, MD, Efstratios Koutroumpakis, MD, Benjamin Click, MD, Marc Schwartz, MD, Jason Swoger, MD, Leonard Baidoo, MD, Jana G. Hashash, MD, Arthur Barrie, MD, Michael A. Dunn, MD, and David G M. Five-year period prevalence and characteristics of anemia in a large U.S. inflammatory bowel disease cohort. Hashash, MD, Arthur Barrie, MD, Michael A. Dunn, MD, and David G M. Five-year period prevalence and characteristics of anemia in a large U.S. inflammatory bowel disease cohort. Physiol Behav. 2016;176(3):139-48.

24. Skikne BS, Punnonen K, Caldron PH, Bennett MT, Rehu M, Gasior GH, et al. Improved differential diagnosis of anemia of chronic disease and iron deficiency anemia: A prospective multicenter evaluation of soluble transferrin receptor and the sTfR/log ferritin index. Am J Hematol. 2011;86(11):923-7.

25. Chang J, Bird R, Clague A, Carter A. Clinical utility of serum soluble transferrin receptor levels and comparison with bone marrow iron stores as an index for iron-deficient erythropoiesis in a heterogeneous group of patients. Pathology. 2007;39(3):349-53.

26. Weiss G, Ganz T, Goodnough LT. Anemia of inflammation. Blood. 2019;133(1):40-50.

27. Beyne-Rauzy O. Inflammatory anaemia: pathophysiology and management.

Rev Med Interne. 2009;30(SUPPL. 4).

28. Yakut M, Üstün Y, Kabaçam G, Soykan I. Serum vitamin B12 and folate status in patients with inflammatory bowel diseases. Eur J Intern Med [Internet]. 2010;21(4):320-3. Available Available from: http://dx.doi.Org/10.1016/j.ejim.2010.05.007

29. Goodhand JR, Kamperidis N, Rao A, Laskaratos F, McDermott A, Wahed M, et al. Prevalence and management of anemia in children, adolescents, and adults with inflammatory bowel disease. Inflamm Bowel Dis. 2012;18(3):513-9.

30. Atul Ö, Kani HT, Banzragch M, Imeryüz N, Akin H. Incidence rate of anemia in inflammatory bowel diseases. Turkish J Gastroenterol. 2016;27(2):143-8.

31. Al-naseem AA, Sallam AA, A ASC, B JT. Iron deficiency without anaemia: a diagnosis that matters. Clin Med (Northfield II). 2021;21(2):107-13.

32. Cacoub P, Choukroun G, Cohen-solal A, Luporsi E. Iron deficiency screening is a key issue in chronic inflammatory diseases: A call to action. J oflnternal Med. 2022;542-556.

33. Herrera-deguise C, Casellas F, Robles V, Navarro E, Borruel N. Iron Deficiency in the Absence of Anemia Impairs the Perception of Health-Related Quality of Life of Patients with Inflammatory Bowel disease. Inflamm Bowel Dis. 2016;22(6):1450-5.

34. Los UMDECDE. WHO guideline on use of ferritin concentrations to assess iron status in individuals and population. 2020.

35. Abitbol V, Borderie D, Polin V, Maksimovic F, Sarfati G, Esch A, et al. Diagnosis of iron deficiency in inflammatory bowel disease by transferrin receptor-ferritin index. Med (United States). 2015;94(26):1-6.

36. Cappellini MD, Comin-Colet J, de Francisco A, Dignass A, Doehner W, S. P. Lam C, et al. Iron deficiency across chronic inflammatory conditions: international expert opinion on definition, diagnosis, and management. Am J Hematol. 2017;92(10):1068-78.

37. Halfvarson J, Cummings F, Grip O, Savoye G, De CHU, et al. Inflammatory bowel disease registries for collection of patient iron parameters in Europe. World J Gastroenterol. 2018;24(10):1063-71.

38. Stein J, Dignass AU. Management of iron deficiency anemia in inflammatory bowel disease - a practical approach. Ann Gastroenterol. 2013;104-13.

39. Goldenberg BA, Graff LA, Clara I, Zarychanski R, Walker JR, Carr R, et al. al. Is iron deficiency in the absence of anemia associated with fatigue in inflammatory bowel disease? Am J Gastroenterol [Internet]. 2013;108(9):1392-7. Available Available from: http://dx.doi.org/10.1038/ajg.2013.14

40. Wozniak M, Baranska M, Malecka-panas E, Talar-wojnarowska R. The prevalence , characteristics , and determinants of anaemia in newly diagnosed patients with inflammatory bowel disease. Gastroenterol Rev. 2019;14(1):39-47.

41. Bielefeldt K, Davis B, Binion DG. Pain and inflammatory bowel disease. Inflamm Bowel Dis. 2009;15(5):778-88.

42. Coates MD, Lahoti M, Binion DG, Szigethy EM, Regueiro MD, Bielefeldt K. Abdominal pain in ulcerative colitis. Inflamm Bowel Dis. 2013;19(10):2207-14.

43. Srinath AI, Walter C, Newara MC, Szigethy EM. Pain management in patients with inflammatory bowel disease: Insights for the clinician. Therap Adv Gastroenterol. 2012;5(5):339-57.

44. Mija DD, Jankovi GLJ, Jorga J, Krsti MN. Nutritional status in patients with active fl ammatory bowel disease: Prevalence of malnutrition and methods for routine nutritional assessment. Eur J Intern Med. 2010;21:315- 9.

45. Julie Rempel KG and WE-M*. Micronutrient Deficiencies and Anemia in Children with Inflammatory Bowel Disease. Nutrients. 2021;5(209).

46. Nguyen GC, Du L, Chong RY, Jackson TD. Hypoalbuminaemia and postoperative outcomes in inflammatory bowel disease: The NSQIP surgical cohort. J Crohn's Colitis. 2019;13(11):1433-8.

47. Rogler G, Vavricka S. Anemia in inflammatory bowel disease: An underestimated problem? Front Med. 2015;2(JAN): 1-8.

48. M. L. Hoivik*,f, W. ReinischJ, M. Cvancarova*,§, B. Moum* & the I study group, *Department. Alimentary Pharmacology and Therapeutics Anaemia in in fl ammatory bowel disease: a population-based. Aliment Pharmacol Ther Anaemia. 2013;(October):69-76.

49. Selinger CP, Parkes GC, Bassi A, Fogden E, Hayee B, Limdi JK, et al. A multi-centre audit of excess steroid use in 1176 patients with inflammatory bowel disease. Aliment Pharmacol Ther. 2017;46(10):964-73.

50. Lee DS, Bang KB, Kim JY, Jung YS, Park JH, Kim HJ, et al. The prevalence and clinical characteristics of anemia in Korean patients with inflammatory

bowel disease. Intest Res. 2016;14(1):43- 9.

51. Frei P, Biedermann L, Nielsen OH, Rogler G. Use of thiopurines in inflammatory bowel disease. World J Gastroenterol. 2013;19(7):1040-8.

52. Hamed KM, Dighriri IM, Baomar AF, Alharthy BT, Alenazi FE, Alali GH, et al. Overview of Methotrexate Toxicity: A Comprehensive Literature Review. Cureus. 2022;14(9).

53. Bedoui Y, Guillot X, Sélambarom J, Guiraud P, Giry C, Jaffar-Bandjee MC, et al. Methotrexate an old drug with new tricks. Int J Mol Sci. 2019;20(20).

54. Magro F, Portela F. Management of inflammatory bowel disease with infliximab and other anti-tumor necrosis factor alpha therapies. BioDrugs. 2010;24(SUPPL. 1):3-14.

55. Dogra S, Khullar G. Tumor necrosis factor-a antagonists: Side effects and their management. Indian J Dermatol Venereol Leprol. 2013;79(SUPPL. 1):35-46.

56. Beaugerie L, Rahier JF, Kirchgesner J. Predicting, Preventing, and Managing Treatment-Related Complications in Patients With Inflammatory Bowel Diseases. Clin Gastroenterol Hepatol [Internet]. 2020;18(6):1324-1335.e2. Available Available from: https://doi.org/10.1016/j.cgh.2020.02.009

57. Torres J, Bonovas S, Doherty G, Kucharzik T, Gisbert JP, Raine T, et al. ECCO guidelines on therapeutics in Crohn's disease: Medical treatment. J Crohn's Colitis. 2020;14(1):4-22.

58. Tim Raine A, Stefanos Bonovas, b, Johan Burisch, c, T orsten Kucharzik D, Michel Adamina, e, Vito Annese F, Oliver Bachmann G, Dominik

Bettenworth H, Maria Chaparro I, et al. ECCO Guidelines on Therapeutics in Ulcerative Colitis: Medical Treatment. J Crohn's Colitis. 2022;17(2).

59. Bergamaschi G, Castiglione F, D'Incà R, Astegiano M, Fries W, Milla M, et al. Prevalence, Pathogenesis and Management of Anemia in Inflammatory Bowel Disease: An IG-IBD Multicenter, Prospective, and Observational Study. Inflamm Bowel Dis [Internet]. 2023 Jan 1;29(1):76- 84. Available from: https://doi.org/10.1093/ibd/izac054

60. Ribiere S, Leconte M, Chaussade S, Abitbol V. Reprint of: Acute severe colitis. J Eur des Urgences Reanim [Internet]. 2018;30(4):146-54. Available from: https://doi.org/10.1016/j.jeurea.2018.10.002

61. Koutroubakis IE, Ramos-Rivers C, Regueiro M, Koutroumpakis E, Click B, Schoen RE, et al. Persistent or Recurrent Anemia Is Associated With Severe and Disabling Inflammatory Bowel Disease. Clin Gastroenterol Hepatol [Internet]. 2015;13(10):1760-6. Available from: http://dx.doi.org/10.1016/j.cgh.2015.03.029

62. S S, Kchir H, Maamouri N, Chaabouni H, Ben MN. Anemia and diseases inflammatory bowel diseases. La Rev m?®decine interne [Internet]. 2016;37:A193. Available from: http://dx.doi.org/10.1016/j.revmed.2016.10.239

TABLE OF CONTENTS